More praise for *Intention Tremor: A Hybrid Collec...*

"*Intention Tremor* is ultimately a book about compassion. Sellman shows us the unseen: the interior experience of living with a stealth disease. I'm grateful for this book for expanded my understanding of a condition I thought I understood."

—Michele Bombardier, author, *What We Do*

"Sellman's intelligence and experience as a prose writer comes through in this hybrid manuscript: poems that bristle with scientific accuracy, prose pieces that border on dreamy intensity and longing."

—Jeannine Hall Gailey, author,
Field Guide to the End of the World

INTENTION TREMOR

Anna
Keep on writing... do it all!,

INTENTION TREMOR
A Hybrid Collection

TAMARA KAYE SELLMAN

Tamara Sellman

Oct 2013

MoonPath Press

Poetry
ISBN 978-1-936657-57-5

Cover photo "Grunge hand (gg4525552)"
by Tawng © www.gograph.com

Author photo by Elizabeth Thorpe

Book design by Tonya Namura using Times New Roman

MoonPath Press is dedicated to publishing the finest poets
living in the U.S. Pacific Northwest.

MoonPath Press
PO Box 445
Tillamook, OR 97141

MoonPathPress@gmail.com

http://MoonPathPress.com

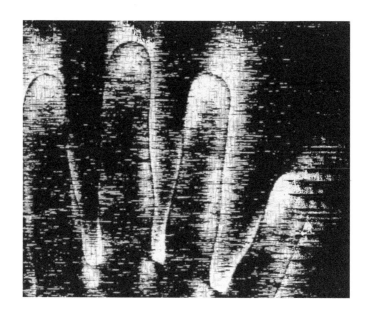

Author proceeds from the sale of this book will be donated to the
Accelerated Cure Project (ACP) (www.acceleratedcure.org).
The ACP's mission: To improve health, healthcare, and quality
of life for people affected by multiple sclerosis (MS)
by connecting those with MS, care partners, clinicians, and
researchers, and to work together to accelerate innovation,
research, and the application of new knowledge.

Acknowledgments

"Diagnosis" previously appeared in *Something on Our Minds* in 2017.

"The Expert" previously appeared in *Halfway Down the Stairs* in 2018.

"Group Admin, Illness Forum" previously appeared in *pioneertown* in 2017.

"Hot Bath Test" previously appeared in *Something on Our Minds* in 2017.

"Kanab" previously appeared in *Cirque* in 2019.

"Map to New Normal" previously appeared in *Snapdragon* in 2019.

"Ouroboros" previously appeared in *Something on Our Minds* in 2015.

"Racer's Edge" previously appeared in *Snapdragon* in 2017.

"Sideways" previously appeared in *Postcard Prose & Poems* in 2018.

"Suddenly, I can't finish my sentences when I try to order Starbucks" first appeared in a slightly different format at *Loud Coffee Press* in January 2020; it was awarded Honorable Mention in the Tom Howard/ Margaret Reid Poetry Contest and reprinted by *Winning Writers* in May 2020.

"Uhthoff's Phenomena" previously appeared in *Barking Sycamores* in 2016, in the 2017 *Barking Sycamores* anthology, and in *The Coil* in 2019.

"Visibility" previously appeared in the *Kissing Dynamite* anthology, "Live Every Voice," in 2019.

"Zebrafish Husbandry" previously appeared in *Blanket Sea* in 2019.

Gratitude

No book happens in a vacuum, and I must give thanks in particular to the following people for supporting my work on this project and out in the world:

To Mike, Amanda, and Megan Sellman, the finest and most creative family one could hope for.

To my second family at Centrum (especially the YAWP): in particular, Michele Bombardier, Wendy Call, Sayantani Dasgupta, Jordan Hartt, and Elizabeth Thorpe.

To my third family at Health Union, especially: Lorene Alba, Alina Ahsan, Tim Armand, Dave Bexfield, Stephanie Buxhoeveden, Olivier Chateau, Cathy and Gary Chester, Shelby Comito, Jennifer and Dan Digmann, Kim Dolce, Lisa Emrich, Noel Forrest, Devin Garlit, Christie Germans, Laura Kolaczkowski, Kerry MacKay, Kelly Miller, Nicole Lemelle, Emily Rhoades, Ashley Ringstaff, Kristin Schwoebel, Kathy Reagan Young, and Kristine Zerkowski.

To the powerful and inspiring writer/activists Glenda Bailey-Mershon, Jen Culkin, Kelly Davio, Yvonne deSousa, Jeannine Hall Gailey, Nicola Griffith, Tara Hardy, Charis Hill, and Alice Wong.

To Deanna Kirkpatrick and Amy Gurowitz for teaching me to laugh at MS. To Stuart Schlossman for his intrepid advocacy. To Janis Segress for showing me what grace looks like. To John Willson for gently prying open my poet's brain. To Kristy Webster for "getting it" on so many levels. To Bill Ransom for confirming it's okay to "just do the thing." To Megan Snyder-Camp for finding the nexus of stars, magic, science, and the ineffable. To Pam Houston for teaching "the 82 percent true memoir."

To my neurologists, Drs. Mariko Kita and Kevin McCarthy, for having my back and listening to me, and to my osteopath Dr. Robert Bethel for being the best doctor I have ever had.

To Lana Ayers, a bottomless thank you for making space for my story, encouraging me to tell it, and really, so much more. Let's get Mora's.

To two unforgettable writers gone from this plane: Waverly Fitzgerald and Jay Lake.

To the arts-savvy Accelerated Cure Project for its ongoing effort to promote the creative work of people with MS.

Finally, to all my chronic peers who have the audacity to rise every day to live their best lives: this world doesn't deserve your infinite light, enduring humor, and rooted strength.

—TKS

Table of Contents

INTENTION TREMOR
A Hybrid Collection

AUGUST 1975

It first happened when she was a month shy of ten. A curly brown ribbon of a girl who played softball, fished for crappie, read books in her cool walkout basement on hot summer days, rode her bike in endless circles. A girl without a stitch of fat, a lean muscular thing flush with the energy that radiated from the ever-curious coals of her brain. A perpetual motion kind of girl, but an obedient girl who rarely asked for attention, who rarely complained of anything except for going to bed at a decent hour.

That day she would pick blackberries in the orchards across the street with one of many best friends named Michelle she would have throughout her life. She laced her shoes, tugged her hand-me-down Wrangler cut-offs into place, grabbed the Tupperware bowl, and stood.

There.

Large grips, stiff and unrelenting, pinched her around the ribcage. She likened them to the curved claws of a 1960s TV show robot. Her fingers fumbled the bowl. It banged in its hollow plastic voice across the wood parquet floor.

Instinctively, she stood even straighter than before, tried to breathe, those intercostal efforts abandoned as the cinching grew severe. Her breaths came shallow, followed by stars in her eyes.

Her grandmother sidled in from the kitchen. *Raise your arms!*

The girl tried to, but the pain seized fresh her ribcage, spasming. Her brown eyes pooled with involuntary tears. She dropped to the floor, a cat on all fours, writhing in the grips of an invisible vice.

As quickly as it had stormed her body, the seizure released. She heaved, young lungs refreshing, tears dropping like rain to dot the squares of yellowed wood around her star-shaped hands. Her mother walked in then, concern in her eyes.

Just a touch of pleurisy, her grandmother said.

SUDDENLY, I CAN'T FINISH MY SENTENCES WHEN I TRY TO ORDER STARBUCKS

—Derived from "Wordfinding Problems and How to Overcome them
Ultimately with the Help of a Computer," Michael Zock, *Proceedings of
the 4th Workshop on Cognitive Aspects of the Lexicon (CogALex)*, 2014

imagine   wishing to   name   'mocha'
                  failing to   find
                           all directly related words

* * *

      (may) I suggest
                a system
                    that accepts whatever
comes to mind   'coffee'
                              'mocha'

* * *

the problem is real
                words are important
                    to meet
                        needs commonly found
in coffee shops

* * *

we want to guess the user's goal
                elusive
                words
           that function like signposts
                      signaling
    the direction to go.
                    reasonable guesses:

      biscuit bitter dark dessert drink cappuccino
        ground   bar   tea   mocha   milk   french
      smell   table   machine   cup   black   beverage
        espresso   pot   cream   house   mud   instant
          strong sugar time break bean morning

say, 'coffee'
'beverage' or 'color' ?
espresso cappuccino mocha
taste food color   target word mocha   evoked term

* * *

lexical access
            involves
                  words meanings forms
                              knowledge of both
agents incomplete

* * *

neither alone
            can point to the target
                        but
                        together
                                    they can.
      as if   one had the map
                        the other
                        a compass

* * *

to find the elusive word   everything being connected
                  is reachable   at least
                        in principle

* * *

he knows   forms   of sound or meaning.
            more general/specific
                        others
                              exactly
                                    the opposite
                        knowledge
so obvious
            so frequent
                        it is encoded (in) the 'relationship'

* * *

(with respect)

he may

provide   the problem

when (s)he cannot access

at this very moment

'tip-of-the-

tongue'

* * *

when looking for   a word,

start from   topology

'black' is related to 'white'

closer than, say,

'black' and 'flower'

* * *

putting words into clusters

is one thing,

naming them…

* * *

it would be nice

to use whatever you have,

incomplete

as it may be

* * *

to help you find what you cannot

one might think of   dark

coffee

beans

Arabia

* * *

a set of candidates ?

arabica, espresso, mocha

COALS

in a circle, glowing red pomegranate seeds,
a random blue flame licking its way through the cracks
of light and dark, tasting the wind for direction.

I poked at the flares, my mind black as the night sky,
I stirred the embers so they could not grow silver
skins. I could not know they were a puzzle to be
solved. Flares and embers in white and black film taken
every six months, with and without contrast dye.

This night, the moon hovers super behind a veil
of preternatural mist, brighter and closer to
the answer than any fire I could ever build.

—dedicated to the Fall 2015 YAWP contingent

WITH ALEXIA WITHOUT AGRAPHIA

—From "Alexia without agraphia in multiple sclerosis," letters to the editor, *Journal of Neurology, Neurosurgery, and Psychiatry*, 1996

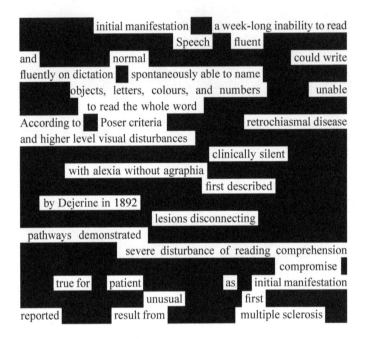

initial manifestation   a week-long inability to read
Speech   fluent
and   normal   could write
fluently on dictation   spontaneously able to name
objects, letters, colours, and numbers   unable
to read the whole word
According to   Poser criteria   retrochiasmal disease
and higher level visual disturbances
clinically silent
with alexia without agraphia
first described
by Dejerine in 1892
lesions disconnecting
pathways demonstrated
severe disturbance of reading comprehension
compromise
true for   patient   as   initial manifestation
unusual   first
reported   result from   multiple sclerosis

DIAGNOSIS

"Here is the proof," Dr. K said, clicking magnetic
scans of my brain, the remarkable white holes,
the countless grains of salt that could grow larger.

"I have a lesion, too," she admitted. "Who
knows how it got there? I'm a neurologist
and I know how it could be anything but."

Except.

In my spinal fluid, cells not normally
invited across that porous aquatic
barrier have left behind their spoor. Over

time and space, narratives in the vault of my
medical records corroborate symptoms—
the tremoring leg, the relentless fatigue,

the crawling skin, the crackling sparklers across
my scalp, the incessant tinnitus, the times
I've left sentences unfinished, don't even

recognize when I have spoken words at all.
Impossible elements in a perfect
cytokine storm. How to right this ship is still

a matter for lab rats, longitudinal
volunteerism, and trial and error.
Choose a new normal. Choose the life of pill bugs.

Or you can choose what's behind door number three.
Her expression was plaintive. What will it be?

Honesty.

She finally smiled, nodded, said,
"Walk heel to toe for me," pointing.
And I did.

DIARY OF A SYNDROME: A hypochondriac's blitz

hiding the truth
hiding a diary
diary in permanent ink

diary of symptoms
symptoms of the brain
symptoms of the body

body of knowledge
body of evidence
evidence of foul play

evidence based
based on opinion
based on facts

facts don't lie
facts on file
file this

file a claim
claim ignorance
claim a dependent

dependent upon circumstances
dependent upon your survival
survival of the fittest

survival story
story structure
story of my life

life force
life with chronic illness
illness and injury
illness and wellness

wellness center
wellness plan
plan for the worst

plan for the unexpected

unexpected company
unexpected pain
pain in the ass

pain management
management of symptoms
management experience

experience setbacks
experience of a lifetime
lifetime warranty

lifetime commitment
commitment heavy
commitment fatigue

fatigue at work
fatigue syndrome
syndrome actor

syndrome or disorder?
disorder?
actor?

FALLEN STARS

There were stars in my mind's sky, and then,
one night, there weren't. Black holes marked
negative silhouettes where astrocytes used to

burn. Even the late August sun lost its radiance
behind filaments of cirrus streaking high in
daylight. We worried: pollution, vitamin D,

rumors of the planet off her poles, if and how
we would survive the fall. When the brain's lights
wink out, when phosphenes curtain vision like

the aurora borealis, you question the pleasure
of staying up to watch the Perseids. Remember
that night? We stretched our bodies across

the bay dock's worn grain, fingers dangling
in bioluminescent tide to conjure manmade
meteor tails. Remember the harmlessness

of shooting stars before diagnosis, how we
saw them first reflected in the bay? When we
looked up, we found the stars first lost to us

by smog returned. My interior galaxy is no more
a marvel: dark stars cluster there now, missing
their points, pressed flat against a matte black

backdrop inside my skull, bathed in a tainted
bay of spinal fluid. I can't connect the junctions
of my brain's star patterns like bookmakers do,

galactic constellations etched, white on blue,
in books: Cygnus, the Dragon, Shield, Northern
Crown. I could hardly find mine, much less

name them, astrocytes that no longer rage white
hot but blink randomly, genetically fueled by
corroded irreplaceable batteries. What I wouldn't

give for a personal Milky Way to brighten my MRI,
its soft glow illuminating the interstitial spaces
of the *corpus callosum*. Soft luminous contrails

to light my way. Instead, mine is a black hole sky
salted in white dots—negative action potentials—
pretending the bravery of five-point stars.

HOT BATH TEST

"For a half century, the hot bath test has been used as a
'diagnostic test' in multiple sclerosis. The appearance
of new neurological signs or aggravation of preexisting
signs generally is transient, with resolution on return of
body temperature to normal. We have observed four
patients...with considerable...prolonged neurological
debilitation after hot bath testing. We suggest caution
in the application of such testing."

—"Persistent neurological deficit precipitated by hot
bath test in multiple sclerosis." *Journal of the American
Medical Association*, May 1983

I didn't know about the test until after diagnosis. Instead,
I was asked to stride a hall, perform touch-your-nose tricks
while standing, eyes closed, flamingo-style, practice
walking on heels like Groucho Marx, then on tippy toes.
Nobody asked me what it's like to take a hot bath. My

thoughts of steaming soaks are linked to Sunday night
memories in childhood. Not forgotten is the sliding into
Avon bubble bath, the persistent tingles, strange itchiness
unrelieved by my ragged tomboy's nails. A weekend's worth
of outdoor grime literally melted from my skin in the suds,

rendering my mother's insistence on washcloth scrubbing
painful and unnecessary. After, I was wrapped in flannel
pajamas before taking in the night's double feature:
Mutual of Omaha's Wild Kingdom opening for *Walt Disney's
Wonderful World of Color*, until Tinkerbell swirled into

the heart of the TV screen, my itching stopped, and I drowsed,
wet hair plastering my chin...   Late in life,
hot baths at bedtime yield similar results. Now I accept that
boiling is not necessary for cleansing, that my speech slurs
after a hard scald like I've drained a bottle of red. Beaujolais

notwithstanding, a bath is not a braise, one's skin should never
cringe and tremble like pale boiled meat. During pregnancy,
I stopped taking soaks out of distrust I might fall standing up
or drown in a faint. Hot showers are no better. My husband
insists the searing blast on the scalp every morning invigorates

as much as a hot cup of coffee. I explain more than once
how it goes for me, how the hotter the water, the more
I'm likely to fall in the battle against the unwelcomed mid-
morning nap, the loss of words paralyzing, the germinating
seeds of migraine wrapped in the stuffy shell of lassitude.

TWO LEFT FEET

See those divots in the brain's
gray and white matter, highlights

in black or white by the
music of magnets and chemo

dye? They're visual skips
from an old record player

used to recite the step-by-steps
in a celestial dance class,

hypo- or hyperintensities
begging attention to footwork

missed in transition. This, the brain
under siege, a place of warped

space-time, a Devil's ballet
debuting the immune system

in unexpected collision with its
central nervous partner.

The production's stellar cast
flashes, clashes inside this

perimetered universe. Cell clusters
struggle with choreography, force

new music, improvisation:
Chopsticks on live piano,

bolts of dubstep, broken harp
strings, vague beatless tracks,

mystery sound effects
(more like a jukebox's

luck of the draw than an
intentional sabotage).

But like the heart, the brain
stores vast collections of

original scores used for self-
correction, protection, redirection

in the face of failed routines
made by any AntiBody.

See how pace, musicality,
time are cited in the program

in the endnotes? Be prepared:
the neural network might

switch production strikes
on lightning feet while

stage directors, in shadows,
plot revisions aloud, pointing:

> *A, you skip B and go to C*
> *instead, and you! C! Join*
> *with F by way of G, and*
> *don't miss your mark!*

(Meanwhile, solo performers,
choose your own adventures

from patterns of floor-
pasted dancing shoes à la

Arthur Miller to best sync
your unique orbits.) Even if

the brain's complex orchestra
fears defeat by clusters of

bad actors hiding behind
red curtains, the show must

go on. Watch the starlet
with two left feet, she

quietly relies on her inner
circle—the *corpus callosum*—

to proffer understudies,
those whose earnest

and anonymous bleeding feet
have memorized every repertoire,

dreaming of grand entrances
in heels that spark comets

like those thrown from Sammy
Davis Jr.'s infamous wingtip taps.

TECFIDERA

I

One. Two. Three. Four. Breathe in. Breathe out. Repeat.
You walk the back road, the trail, the high school track,

take the stairs two by two, arms attuned to hips in motion,
warm, loose and fluid, controlled. Fingers tingle, balance

veers always to the left, your ears filled with tinnitus opera.
The crown of your head tilts, spilling the leftover fairy dust

of chi from the nape of your neck. Always, there is extra,
the spoils of energy gained, then lost in the act of living.

II

The commercial shows a woman who is you, but you are
not an actor. She moves through the acts of her life:

in Spring, striding as a speedwalker; in Summer, diving
into the blue of a pool, crawling stroke over stroke to

the other side; then, in the Autumn, riding a Ferris wheel
at the county fair. A man in the hovering bench next to her

brandishes the turquoise capsule: Elixir of Tecfidera,
a diamond ring for her to swallow at the top of the carnival.

III

Each dose more than a hundred dollars. Twice a day, every
day. The promise to stay the march of T cells consuming

the memory of muscle, the glimmer of crystalline thought,
the music of speech, all that is you, without discrimination.

You gird yourself with fried eggs, tuna fish in oil, bananas
and peanut butter at every meal to coat your gut so you can

swallow chemotherapy whole, survive its secondary insults
in order to take your walk, climb your stairs, live your life.

IV

Today it is stadium steps, cold gray concrete. *Two by two,
breathe in, breathe out.* Your body a metronome tuning

its efforts to thwart the random violence of astrocytes
turned against you, chiseling, faceting, cauterizing both

the white matter and the gray. Moving the body mobilizes
blood factors, strengthens the myelin sleeves of neurons,

feeds oxygen to the factories of the mitochondria, makes
efficiency of glucose so your brain doesn't trip its circuits.

V

The chipped amber paint on the edge of each step evokes
that first week of track season every year in high school.

Shin splints and Icy Hot. Paced breathing to fuel muscles.
This was decades ago, but just last night you dreamed of

running. The air inside your lungs didn't burn. Your muscles
like soft pulled taffy, your gait a weightless dance of

forward motion. Today, you try to run. Footfalls wobble,
threaten to shatter in seconds your contractured ankles.

VI

The promise of a pill. Many tolerate it less than the daily
bee stings administered at one of seven injection sites,

tattoos using needles dripping the ink of recombinant DNA.
You covet your capsule, your personal Hope Diamond.

Three years now, you've since become the pill popper
the small-town grocery clerk disparaged while ringing up

your soy milk. Her cure for everything is your poison, says
your apologetic naturopath. *Breathe in, breathe out.*

JOHN CUNNINGHAM LIVES

"John F. Cunningham was a patient at the VA Hospital in Wood,
Wisconsin, in the summer of 1970. Cunningham had Hodgkin's disease
and 'rather rapidly progressing neurologic deficits.' He was given a
diagnosis of PML* during life on the basis of a brain biopsy and thereafter
'expressed the wish that his brain should aid research into this fatal disease.'
A 'new human polyoma virus' was subsequently detected by [co-discoverer
Dr. Gabriele M. Zu] Rhein and her colleagues in Cunningham's postmortem
brain tissue, and the virus was named JC virus in honor of the patient."
—from Pathophilia: *For the Love of Disease*, January 23, 2012

Dear John

You are in our cells, our thoughts, our cerebrospinal fluid, a host
virus that haunts the chosen few. This is the way it always is…not
everyone who enters a haunted house will see a ghost, even when the
spirits come down from the attic to throw parties that linger late at the
kitchen table, leaving behind toast crumbs.

You don't mind being rejected by us. You get it. You would hate
yourself too, if you knew what had gotten into you. You linger in at
least half of all of us, often dormant for a lifespan, but sometimes the
conditions of mitochondria achieve a vortex, and there you are, the one
we get to blame.

Like most of us, you didn't choose your end except to share what
little was left of you. Bits of gray matter extracted, smudged against
slides, cultured to curate what would become the discovery of a new
intracellular virion. In a sense, your identity wasn't alive to us until
well after you'd died.

Your act of leaving became, ironically, a permanent earthbound
stay defined by your acronym. JCV, with PML riding shotgun: dark
partners to interrogate under naked lightbulbs. Because we broke you,
we now know one way to retard the curse of unintended consequences.

My friend Jay gifted his genome to science to discover why cancer
loved him so much. I still shed tears for the cross sections of Lucy at
Chicago's Museum of Natural History. Henrietta Lacks didn't have
a choice, hers a theft of mother culture by the privileged of the ivory
tower, yet birthing a new paradigm of consent. Life in spite of death.

I do wonder…do you ever look back and find you rue your gift, wish instead to leave behind something other than the vector of a rare brain infection? Would you apologize to those with AIDS, to organ transplant patients, for riding roughshod over their immune systems?

You shouldn't. Because you let us peek under your hood, we know now what to look for when we peek under our own. I'm glad with every six-vial blood draw taken every three months to find you haven't dropped your inner tube into my bloodstream. You, the hero I hope to never meet.

* PML: Progressive multifocal leukoencephalopathy (PML) is a dangerous viral brain infection that targets the cells which make myelin, the insulated coating of nerve cells.

PILL POPPER AT THE BLUE STAR DINER

My meds popped out of their case, diverse
escapees shaped as capsules, tablets,
gel caps in orange, white, pink, brown,
or teal for the known furniture biocide
I take twice daily at one hundred

bucks a pop. Drugs scatter across the
classic diner countertop—turquoise
formica topped with fading golden
starlights—or they wobble, full of oil.
Some are, thankfully, flat and resigned

to the fact of recapture. As I scoop up
what I've come to call fondly
a Second Breakfast—a dozen plus
therapeutic agents my neuro
calls a cocktail—I miss the tiny

chalk wheel of vitamin D as it
plunges to the filthy diner floor.
I shrug. At pennies on the dollar,
it can be missed, and I plan to see
the sun later anyway. Meanwhile,

others stare from behind club sandwich
bites or forkfuls of fried eggs, the slight
narrow of their eyes defining me
an outlier for packing drugs as if
I'm an addict or raging hypochondriac.

RACER'S EDGE

My friend, when I told her my fate, wept
like a funeral mourner, her tears
a puzzling death sentence.

How *am I?*

Maybe a better question is, *where* am I?

I am here, in front of you, corporeal,
speaking, walking, alert and alive.

I could be home on the couch wrapped in paralysis.
I could be stuck with needles in an infusion ward
soaking up chemo. I could have wheels for feet.
I could be wordless and drooling, incapable of
swallowing, a hypersomniac, incontinent.

Instead, I am having lunch with you.

The spectrum of where I now live, surveyed
by a standard index, places me just paces
beyond the starting line, nowhere near the tape
at the end of a race I never plan to finish.

Don't wait for me there at the end.
I am not a ghost, not any more than you are.

THE EXPERT

sits online, overstimulated by blue spectrum light, scouring for
evidence, though all he understands is purely anecdotal. The first-
person accounts, the stories from a friend of his sister's boyfriend's
boss. He misinterprets clinical studies, decides two and two equal five,
wonders why science is taking so long to discover a capital C cure.

He is not a biologist, but he might be a theologist. He does not know *B
cells* from *jail cells* from *T cells* from *killer cells* from *supercells*. He
thinks the cure is known, locked in a cylinder in a vault in Antarctica
where nobody will ever find it except through an act of espionage.

He thinks sick people are the cash cows of the Corporation. That
vaccines are for fools. That medicine is poison, Big Pharma the enemy.
But vitamins are miracles, even when they cost you your electric bill,
and if you drank special water, ate special diets, performed special yoga
poses, the gut biome would reverse itself and eliminate your (dis) ease.

Our web evangelizer believes you will fall for his friendly profile
picture, the posts about his dogs, his misspelled words and conspiracy
theories posted at hours when only insomniacs breed. Who knows who
he really is? To be sure, we could all stand to look in the mirror to see
who we are and who we are not.

LASSITUDE

Daily I wake up, consult
my toes and head, then spin the
Wheel of Fortune, determine

the day's journey for that first
foot on soft carpet. Some days
the pointer lands on the bright

green pie shape. I take its lead
and hike in the forest. When
it chooses the crimson pie

wedge, I drink extra water,
take all my meds, welcome naps,
practice self-preservation

by way of mindless housebound
domestic chores if only
to feel productive between

random dizzy spells and pain.
I still prefer this outcome
to the steel blue triangle

at pointer's end. Its only
promise is systemic dread.
To lift or not lift myself

out of the comfortable crypt
that is my bed? The gut gnaws,
insists that it is better

to eschew living entire
days I have yet to enter
properly, a seductive

lie which easily renders
surrender flags from bedsheets
still warm from the night, even

as heart and mind bear witness
and protest potential falls
not caused by failing ankles.

SIDEWAYS

Yesterday I woke up sideways. Descending the stairs,
I used the railings without white knuckles—I don't fear

new adventures anymore. My eyes cocked 45 degrees,
left of center, even when the crown of my head pointed

straight up to the chakra constellations that orbit there,
invisible. *Do my eyes look funny?* I asked him.

He shook his head. *Is my mouth drooping?* He answered No.
Am I walking a straight line? My eyes, at slant, noted

the floor, found no evidence of ersatz gravity,
which I assumed would be the natural outcome of life

on the diagonal. *You look fine to me*, he said,
so I sat at my desk and got to work on deadlines.

INTENTION TREMOR

The gate agent at LaGuardia informs me of storm-related flight cancellations, gives me a false-lashed stink eye as I take my new boarding pass, fingers quaking uncontrollably.

It's not that bad. The gate agent's eyes roll.

Listen, I want to tell her, *if my flight had been early, if I was already home and not completely exhausted, my hands would still be doing this.*

It's a muscle puzzle my brain can't solve. My hands hang forgotten at my side until I reach for a cup of coffee, brace myself against a chair rail, or lift fingers to push curls from my brow. There it is: the intention tremor. At least my hands twang painlessly, like bass guitar strings pulled too tight. But for the weakness of my wrists, all the dropped coffee cups, I might not even mind it.

In the plane aisle, I can't convince the nearby attendant that I need assistance raising my carry-on to stow above my seat. My hands' relentless jitterbug makes grasping even the lightest thing an illusion.

I'm sorry, we can't help you, the flight attendant tells me through sour pink lemonade lipstick,

We can only help those who are actually disabled.

When you hear that enough times, you like to believe you become desensitized to it.

The involuntary fidget in my upper thigh joins in the dance then, choreographed to the rattle of leg muscles which can't help but spasm in such tight, inflexible quarters. Experience warns me: if I reach up, I will surely lose balance and coordination.

Simmer down, I silently command my postural tic, laughing at the impossibility. If I could only sit down. Instead, I'll probably fall down.

What I recall more vividly than my insensitive hosts, however, is the traveler in the cross-aisle seat. Faceless and not particularly gallant or chivalrous. A man more interested in his smartphone, who assists me without a word. A man who doesn't need to see a doctor's note.

UHTHOFF'S PHENOMENA

There is a sun in my head. A dark star
sun. No blinding rays to shoot through ears, eyes
and nostrils, just potential heat stored in
Uhthoff's famous furnace, waiting for a
cerebral match to trigger the pilot.

A hot shower can boil my internal
sun into being. To avoid stoking
new wildfires, I can only use the cold
setting on my blow dryer. If I am
cooking or baking, I have to open

the windows. Hot weather calls for dwelling
in shade, charging portable fans, packing
ice, spraying my skin with menthol, quaffing
pitchers of cold drinks to cool down my core.
Even on freezing winter days, hidden

heat ignited by my sun forces my
coat's return to the closet and a crank
on the AC in the car. When my star
blooms, my skull sweats from the inside, a warm
oily wash across the dura, trickling

through the weave of the *corpus callosum*,
until it reaches muscle fibers, lymph
and arterials. I feel the star's dark
new pulse as it spreads its hot lava flood
every time I try to find words. Nonsense

slurs from my lips, delayed by the struggle
to recall children's names, cell phone numbers,
how to spell the word *The*. Meltdown evokes
a roaring tinnitus concert; even
the thrumming acoustics of MRI

cannot cancel out this racket. Meanwhile,
I will into life conscious breathing, think
through each step needed to walk five feet,
forget how to count my change at Safeway
because trust in strangers is easier.

To put the fire out, I succumb to naps,
wait for my star to burn itself to ash,
let the brain send crews to survey damage,
launch its post-trauma restoration opps,
and pick through the rubble for survivors.

KANAB

I want to go to Kanab. Dry and red,
hot and lost, a place of high-noon distress.

There I could be a hermit, I could build
a kiva, disguise it with sagebrush, sink
into its cool shade, stare down scorpions—
anything to silence words and voices.

At least you don't have cancer.

At least it won't kill you.

Instead my days are links in an endless
chain of rain, moss, and MRIs…blood draws,
talk of the risks of immunomodulators,
guerilla approaches to side effects.

My speech—already compromised by a
broken brain—fails new vocabulary
lists: *paresthesia, gadolinium,
Lhermitte's, neurological pruritis.*

Meanwhile I can still pronounce *geoduck.*
Kinnick kinnick. Aurora borealis. Sequim.

My old self at diagnosis was tossed
like a broken mannequin into the
salal-ridden ditch of lost identities, not by
a careless doctor or a cruel nurse,

but by those who I expected to know
better than to lob trite comparisons.

Chronic autoimmune disease, without
a cure or even an understanding
of root cause, is no better or worse than
any cancer or other protracted
death. It's the devil of uncertainty
which unites us all, indiscriminate.

At least you don't have cancer.

At least it won't kill you.

What do these words even mean?

I know what *drizzle* means, and
high slack tide, Old Man's Beard.

I remain on the island, damp and green,
cool and contained, a place of hard-pan clay.

I hear the voices in the fog, find their
clever words veiled in the constant
and unlikely solace of tinnitus.

The joints of failing alder trees
pop against autumn's gusts, promising
widowmakers hidden in the furred
and widespread arms of cedar.

This is no Kanab, but I will make do.

THE WORDS, BUT FOR THE WORDS

"But the fear, the grief, the rage…those are the province of cancer and its bubble, shared down to the bone and soul by others in their same bubbles.

"Surely this is true of AIDS, or diabetes, or multiple sclerosis. Surely every sufferer carries their own bubble. Cancer is not special."
—Jay Lake, *The Specific Gravity of Grief*

It's been seven years since Jay died, and I have deep cleaned my office three times since.

I don't mind dusting off his ghosts. Or his memoir, left on my nightstand, waiting for its moment to haunt me in a more subversive way.

I was going to give his book away once I finished it. A slim, 82 percent true memoir about his life enduring four separate turns with malignancy. Colon first, then lungs second and third, then prostate. After his memoir was published, he had one more round of colorectal cancer before June 1 liberated him five days shy of his fiftieth trip around the sun.

* * *

I held on to the artifacts from his weekend-long wake in Portland, the one he organized and attended, though he hobbled on tenterhooks in the fancy socks I gave him to help soften his steps. We smiled and gazed across the rented room filled with revelers drinking to their inspirations, but barely spoke because…words.

Hundreds of friends and fans had collected to auction off the stuff from his basement to raise money against the rising cost of his metastasis. I walked away with baseball and Pinewood Derby trophies from 1970s Taiwan, a funky cogs-in-motion wall clock that now resides on my daughter's wall, an old school phone charger straight out of Ma Bell land.

* * *

He and I used to have small, intense conversations about losing words. Or not finding them. Or having to learn how to smoke them out by other means when our neural pathways developed potholes—his from chemo, mine from demyelination.

He loved it that I referred to these armor chinks as potholes. He loved it that I found strange comfort in solving Sudoku problems, that I saw in numbers a kind of language and logic that words did not possess. That my brain, like his, seemed to demand new ways to process ideas when the old ways had failed.

But for the words. We'd dipped our feet, our entire lives, in the same well, walked in those story spaces between the real and the imagined even before meeting at that science fiction convention ten years before.

The last time we spoke, it was at another convention at SeaTac, and he shared the story of mapping his genome with my daughter—the same age as his daughter—when he discovered she was interested in genetics.

Hope is a reconnaissance unit always scouting new ways in.

* * *

There are always battles at hand in the world of creative writing. Who can write what? When is realism not? Who deserves recognition? For both of us, the time for glancing blows against these privileges dissolved in the moments of diagnosis.

Instead, we fought for the privilege of having access to language at all, using our words as arsenals when we could, to say what others cannot.

It wasn't until I put down his memoir that I realized he'd acknowledged me; he'd bestowed upon me the honor of caption head for the chronically ill in the early pages of his memoir. I had no idea I'd been promoted to this level almost three years before, when he was yet alive, and given new papers to fight against the cold, invisible war against disease we'd both endured.

It mattered not that we had incongruent prognoses. We'd negotiated these same potholes together, wary of mines, mortar, and the myriad ways in which we didn't get to choose.

I cannot give it away now, not this copy. His words have become my manifest. The ink on the page, my orders, still bleed on the page where he signed his name.

THE *N*TH HALF-YEARLY MRI

Radiology techs wrap my feet in shapeless sheaths with rubber skids.
Swaddle me, neck to toe, in thin cotton blankets: a hospital's
sarcophagus. Insert an IV for the contrast session. Shroud my eyes with
a folded washcloth, crown me with earphones playing barely perceived
music to prevent hearing damage.

Please, no more damage.

The exposed top of my head will be sliced by invisible magnetic forces
into pictures.

MRI was first used to investigate the brains of people with lesion
activity seven years after my first MS hug. Those inaugural scans took
five hours. Mine will take 90 minutes.

After the techs' retreat to a control deck behind heavy glass, I am
interred into the narrow tube, asked to lay motionless while drums bang
strange patterns that I find—oddly— rhythmic enough to fall asleep to.

Magnetic resonance is now familiar territory, removing my need for a
lorazepam refill.

This is not death.

Forty-five minutes pass in perfect stillness superimposed over the
spasming kink in my back.

After, they draw me from my high-tech tomb, unravel one edge of my
mummy's wrap near the thigh, prick the IV to start the gad-dye drip,
send me back for a second harvest.

Contrast session. The burn in the veins. *It is so hot in here.*

Finally, they extract me from the tube, the IV pulled out, the wraps
lifted.

Sitting exposed in the cold, dark room, my senses reassert themselves.
Cells expand, breathe, jump, squall like newborn babies clearing their
lungs.

I can't wait— still can't wait, at age 52—to get up and walk away from these compassionate, if anonymous keepers, to leave the hospital's familiar maze, hike the dirty city streets downhill to my ferry ride home to New Normal because, at least, on this rainy spring day, I can.

THE YEAR I CAME HOME FROM THE WAR

followed three years spent grieving fresh diagnosis.
During my time in those trenches, a bloodless coup
commenced, cold and indifferent. My gray matter
callused. My stomach shredded and relined itself.
The ringing in my ears roared despite the silence

of it all. Later, the flash grenades I'd lobbed at
robot insurers and ignorant minions of
Dr. Google were the same hot potatoes that
blasted me a path to my New Normal after
MS reassigned my orders. In peace time, I'm

a civilian now, and yet my war wounds persist—
surprise attacks of nerve pain across dermatomes,
the sabotage of my vitality by an
unseen enemy, the inactive lesions and
distressing side effects of medications. When

symptoms re-emerge, I perform reconnaissance
missions to rule out foreign invaders. There is
no such thing as diplomacy in this cold war,
nor should you call me a warrior. In spite of
the armor of my intellect, which I've used to

forge words into worthless ballistics, I did not
volunteer to become a veteran of this
exhausting assault on my spirit. If you catch
me looking over my shoulder, I'm not looking
for a fight, but for reasons not to fight at all.

CROSSWORD CLUE: ROAD TO A CURE?

It's been an icy, salt-layered winter; an early spring's hot sun has fissured the surfaces of the city's roads.

Imagine a short street, a half-block linkage inside a city's transportation grid. We stand on Axon Street, its concrete cracked into stars under the fat waddle of truck treads, potholes filled with gravel scooped from suburban highway depots. Even if Axon Street is insignificant, it's still a road citizens hypothetically expect to ferry traffic from A to B.

But let's pause. Reimagine.

When you think of tiny Axon Street, envision a nerve cell in your brain. Not one of the main nerves with its own name, not the body-long root connecting crown to sole (soul?). It's just another tiny junction. But, like the street itself, it has potholes of its own.

Neurologists call them *lesions*. But *pothole* works, though these are no humble ruts in the Axon Street-slash-nerve cell, but crumbled hollows sprawled, seeking to gain ground across the adjacent sidewalk egress, too hazardous to cross, threatening sinkholes. Trucks along our metaphoric Axon Street avoid them altogether or risk damaging their undercarriages. Those on foot spy the hazard from the corner, consider ankle sprains, broken heels, stubbed toes, take the next street.

With humble Axon Street at an impasse, the brain—the city—suffers. Traffic jams, commuter complaints of lost time, more gas to burn. Holding the purse, it is the Mayor who reminds us: *Everything costs. It's only one street.* Until it's not.

It's been an icy, salt-layered winter; four new byways reveal fresh erosion—Synapse Avenue, Dendrite Way, the Road of Ranvier, Glial Lane. Commuter hours fall to gridlock, yet Hizzoner worries about votes lost in election-year sinkholes, a budget that needs seal-coating.

Beneath the skim of city politics, broken arterials confirm immune system attacks to the axon's waxy myelin skin. When the brain attempts to conduct electrical signals across a neural network made ragged with potholes, that's the harsh winter of demyelination: it halts, delays, detours neurons. Signals are lost or made late to scheduled appointments with virtually every bodily function (thinking, breathing, speaking, shitting).

Meanwhile, back in our hypothetical brain-slash-city, it's the Fire Department acting on fresh damage because SAFETY FIRST. They contract the brain's own road crew which, using gifts of time and space, remyelinates its own network via organic technology. A new contract—Anti-LINGO 1*—could free up new repair crews if only the mayor valued sustainable budgets. If only.

Instead, Axon Street gets typical Band-aid triage—buckets of asphalt, dump trucks brimming with gravel, Streets & Sanitation's annual patchwork parade in the spring, complete with its merry troupe of Dayglo orange vests and clinking shovels.

City flow is restored, if only because red letter days loom large. Until those ballots are cast, the mayor transfers monies, discredits editorials about too much roadwork.

Election Night eve brings reports that City Hall has brokered back-door deals with union giant Corpus Callosum, a move about as efficient as driving from LA to NYC because planes aren't yet refueled. *It will bring jobs!* sez the Mayor, though we know this is only busywork to enable the electorate.

Welcome to Healthcare by Committee, an era of bottomless taxpayer-funded feasibility studies, the improbable promises of traffic-calming measures, data for data's sake. Axon Street & Friends flyers now herald the formation of potluck vigils for moments when intersections crumble under surface stress and people die.

Now, skip to the future: Mayors, routes, neighborhoods, budgets, priorities may change, but asphalt and gravel come as predictable as the wave of third shift workers who clock in every April, tilting steaming shovels of cement and stone into the hungry mouth of the 5am frost, unaware they're embedding the word *cure* into fresh aggregate: black tar and false hope.

Yes, it's been an icy, salt-layered winter, but I am still here, and I still need flat pathways to span the tiniest potholes.

Anti-LINGO 1 (aka opicinumab) is a potential treatment for MS that promotes remyelination of damaged nerves.

QUARANTINE

begins between Halloween
and Veterans Day after
my flu inoculation.
Safeway grocery shopping

happens after 8pm
or not at all, bottle of
hand sanitizer in my
pocket for times when the store

supply disappears. Wearing
a face mask doesn't really
protect me from the hacking
up of lungs and other fine

particles that people seem
happy to share with neighbors.
I reserve these for plane trips
made necessary by work

interests, hoping to send
a message of awareness.
I have been lucky so far;
head colds that last 14 days,

the feels-like-Norovirus
GI tract disruptions more
likely related to meds,
but no real influenza.

Immunocompromised, I
belong to that exclusive
club filled with babies and old
people, defending against

that much larger club who fears
the modern miracles of
vaccines, eschewing science,
praising herd immunity. I'm

no germaphobe, this is no
hypochondriac's fable.
I've been told *Don't risk it* by
more than one physician. My

DMTs render blood test results
that mirror the compromise of
AIDS, so I choose quarantine to
survive six months of other

people's freedom of choice.
Yes, they're out there, and they're
deadly. People with MS die
from smaller things, after all,

like hospitalization for UTIs
the healthy cavalierly fend off
with glasses of cranberry juice.
The days dawn dark until March,

prompting morning rituals
with Happy Light and coffee
cup. I can't take vacations
from Facebook lest I lose touch

with people who care, ponder
the simple gift of having
a husband who looks forward
to daily grocery trips.

*Note: I wrote this poem in 2016, long before the COVID-19
pandemic. Most immunocompromised people must self-
quarantine during flu season or they risk flareups and
infections that can potentially lead to hospitalization and may
result in death. This, and falls, are the chief ways that people
with MS die from their disease.*

OUROBOROS

The way of multiple sclerosis parallels the stealth of a boa constrictor—muscular, quiet, hidden, coiled around one's brain, opportunistic for the moment it can slide in and swallow your nervous system, part by part, in one long, slow digestive assault.

You try to avoid stress, that favored mantra from the neurologist's office rendered useless in the face of real life—a series of nothing but stressful events linked by rare pauses in space and time, if one is lucky enough to enjoy the luxury of remission.

People die, in real life. You received the news in a text from your brother just minutes ago. Your mother has died, her brain intact, unlike yours, her body riven by crippling arthritis. Awake, conscious, she succumbed when the morphine exceeded her ability to breathe, and suffocated.

As you surely will do here, in this feed store, despite its high hay lofts and capacity to house a circus.

* * *

You tell yourself it is allergies that knot your throat, though you are only sensitive to chemicals and not the floating fibers of straw, the underlying notes of manure. The feed store is a converted barn much larger on the inside than it appears from the road. So much like the lives of the chronically ill.

You've come here with her before, to buy cheap pansies and rubberized garden gloves, to pick up your weekly CSA share. The feed store was then, and is still today, a place for breathing, wide open double-high rafters, light shafting through windows open to the sun and bees in reconnaissance, a place bearing the images held close to your mother's from life grown up on a dairy farm.

To think your mother died because she could no longer breathe—despite the longevity of her lung cancer survival at over twenty years—seems improbable. Maybe she, too, carried a secret snake coiled in her chest in hibernation. She had two aunts and two cousins with MS.

Wrapping your brain and heart around this sudden news renews in you fears both old and recent. It took you years to learn to breathe underwater; only at age forty did you master it without holding your nose. And the small confinements of your new normal after diagnosis? They never bothered her like they bother you now—the tube of the MRI still requires lorazepam, a washcloth over the eyes, a mother's swaddling.

You are not sure you will ever get used to any of this.

On the bench next to you are packets of bulbs, a mulching fork, a bag of hummingbird nectar you can no longer give to her. You hold your breath, hoping the snake doesn't notice. After all, even though you once feared suffocation, your bigger fears, every day, twine around the potential loss of the eyes, the legs, the bladder. Ironically, never the lungs.

* * *

It will hit you later, the way your body will absorb this stress, this loss, like poison. The way the boa constrictor waits for the chemical imbalance to unravel nerve fibers, to send inflammation as a flood of tenderizing blood to repair what cannot be fixed.

And behind the rush of this pointless healing: the yawning pink maw of the snake, its only goal to feed on broken places, digesting them whole with potent enzymes in a process stretched over weeks, leaving irreparable the bare spots, the lost functions.

The boa constrictor moves a third of a mile an hour, the same speed in which you process the news now and for months after, grief presenting as the vice-like squeeze around the rib cage, called an MS hug, not at all alike the one you wish you could give your mother now.

GROUP ADMIN, ILLNESS FORUM

I found my sublet online one day while in my pajamas, my muscles too stiff to move, the shower too hot to tolerate. I was taken in like a rain-drenched stranger on a cold November night. Somebody dried my clothes, I was given a robe and towels, a stein of hot cocoa appeared near a blazing fire that warmed the whole flat. The walls were thick, the floors layered in rich animal skins or exotic woven rugs. At first, I didn't stray from the luxury of the sitting room, but finally I did, and discovered it was a castle. Though there were a few rats inside the walls, the well water sometimes needed boiling and the windows were painted shut, I decided to stay.

I strolled from room to room, discovered beautiful broken people who sang of loss, love and adventure. I pried razors from shaking fingers, handed out butterscotches, became a translator once I mastered house dialect. Two years later the landlords gave me keys to the vault. Deputized, I found a compassionate end for the rats, hired a plumber, stripped down and cranked open the windows to release years of stagnation. I wasn't alone; others baked pies, polished the banister of their own free will. One played the parlor harpsichord deftly. Another donned jester's points and told stories on the parquet floor in bell-tipped shoes.

But there were others, who painted obscenities in India ink on the hallway wallpaper. Collectors of flying termites and black widow spiders. Wailing women with skin so transparent we weren't convinced they weren't already ghosts, encumbered by worldly pain. There were naughty children who told fibs at the dinner table and elderly matriarchs who poked you with the sharp ends of their canes if you came within distance, and sometimes the noise level vibrated the crown molding and sent cracks across the plaster ceiling and we would have to send everyone back to their rooms in order to sweep up and patch and sand ourselves back into normalcy.

When somebody passed, we were elegant in our sobriety. There was never a formal ceremony, only gossip leading to prayers and embraces, soft words spun of the silk of truth, heads nodding, eyes clear and long sighs heard in tandem. We are more than our bodies, so we left the burials of us to the skilled sexton who lived quietly in the white cottage out back. Inside, windows were thrust open even to the rain, and we tipped crystal flutes of crisp cider to salute the dead around a dining room table void of fruit, because who could eat? All of us looking at every other one of us, knowing, and yet, wondering…when?

—*dedicated to Amy, Deanna and Stuart*

VISIBILITY

shines light on the monster in the corner,
prepares us for the grief that comes after
the loss that hasn't happened yet, but will.

The parts of its body are not monstrous,
there is no freakish extremity to chronic,
incurable illness. Giving one's silhouette

a name, a face, an outline, color and texture
is not an act of surrender, but ownership.
Sometimes, the greater miscreation is

the one unseen even when the sun is zenith
high. To put pen to paper, voice to mic,
needle to corpse may appear to animate

atrocity, but let's remember: Frankenstein
was a doctor first, a mortal who cowered
in shadows, summoning lightning bolts

for illumination because the privileged
refused to invest in more humane inquiry.
We are left to the piecework of calamities—

stitching arm to shoulder, knee to shin,
lash to lid, heart to breastbone—wrapping
ourselves in fabric dyed by tears, shed

in secret, to flesh out worst-case scenarios.
This is not abomination, but permission to
persist. We are not vectors; the reservoir

of our mortality can no more be blamed on
failures in personal virtuosity than long life
can be credited for intentional acts of biology.

So cast your deeper, darker shade upon us,
but let's not forget: Frankenstein was a
doctor first, a monster only second born.

MAP TO NEW NORMAL

may look like a highway lined with the signs of the past
but let's not confuse the memory of the Before

with the unknown of the After. Diagnosis puts
an address for a cul-de-sac on the map, that's all.

I am there sleeping between peeks at cartographies
drafted and given to me by friends and strangers who

know the switchbacks, roadblocks, construction sites, duck
crossings, speed traps, parade delays and black ice ahead.

Who takes this highway without realizing possibility?
Who only finds travel guidance in the rearview mirror?

How can they not become lost forever? My doctor
says I've been wandering blind this side road for maybe

as long as forty years, blindly living random fate
like anyone else, never spotting intersections where

odd numbers of streets meet at angles—hallowed ground
where curses and miracles are born only to be

abandoned in litters. I was a working mother: life
equaled exhaustion. Yes, sometimes the afflicted

drive these streets to their graves having never known
they were ever sick. The chaos of living life built of

plans and passion can be just the right distraction
for hurling oneself through traffic circles of pain, distress,

brokenness. It took me decades to trace the paths of
back-to-back infections, strange speech pathologies,

memory blots at age twenty five, roadside naps at
commuter hour before I finally took a closer look.

These maps unfolded across the hood of my car mark
the same throughways, but in changing topography,

ley lines that require diverse access points, different
modes of transportation, even if none of us can

choose our own adventures across these roads leading to
anywhere and yet nowhere at all. Am I travel-

worthy? For now, my body is imprecise but intact,
my brain's neural network of overpasses, side roads

and major arterials only slightly ravaged by potholes
of demyelination. I take heart that U-turns, express lanes,

tunnels and detours remain likely options, that if given time,
a road crew might yet arrive to fill those grooves with

steaming black asphalt. Don't cry for me because I
know something more about myself today than I did

only yesterday. Don't cry for my aunt, who spent her life
mangled in a wheelchair before modern medicine labeled

MS by its cellular pedigree. Don't cry for the cousin who was
given a cane and a prayer in the pre-Google age. Don't cry

for friends who've raised kids to healthy adulthoods, who
still rise daily with sight, mobility, just enough fuel for

the trip to work. They've already found the milestone
I'm only finding for the first time—the exit from

Old normal to New, a bypass lined with orange cones
to mark freshly painted shoulders. I dream of the day

I can access my disease by private lane like they do,
my name on the green reflective sign planted perpendicular

to meet the rest of the world. Today I hunt that property.
I choose the map of watercolors, start the day with a pot

of joe, my brightest lamps to cut the shadows, road trip
music to drown out the tinnitus, an endless sky

for my horizon. Rest stops, scenic routes, festivals
and roadhouses pop up where only my people dance.

ZEBRAFISH HUSBANDRY

"Hey guys super genius in daylight eggs and fertilized it and I have the
eggs and they're going to hatch suit and if you like this video please give it
a thumbs up and if you're new to my channel please subscribe thanks" [sic]
    —YouTube: "zebra danio eggs" uploaded by Feeling Fishy on
      June 9, 2017.

I watched the boy talk about his aquarium on YouTube. He was a
scruffy one, all bedhead and unabashedly honest about the fact he was
not great at making videos.

His handheld camera shots made me queasy. His dead-air pauses
would have been awkward had the boy not been charming to watch as
the cogs whirled in his head, his unmade bed in the background
confirmation he was human in his chaos.

His chief male zebrafish was named Luke, and when he talked
about how the adults eat their young, he paused again, performed a
brief ceremony, his version of Taps.

This is the face of young science.

"That's how random I am," he says in the video. "I see random
things."

* * *

So did George Streisinger.

The University of Oregon researcher got tired of not being able to
see inside the brains of mice.

This was in the 1960s, mind you, before the MRI was invented, a
tool meant primarily to look at the brains of people with demyelinating
disease.

Streisinger went down to the local pet store and bought himself a
tankful of zebrafish. How random is that?

I wonder if Dr. Streisinger had an aquarium as a child. How else
might he have known about these amazing invisible fish and their
accidental window into the biology of the human brain?

You'll have to ask the divine if this discovery truly was an accident.

* * *

It wasn't until after the turn of the 21st century that zebrafish became famous for their biological applications.

Whodathunk? A stunning debut in *Glia**.

Maybe the boy in the YouTube video already knew this. He talks about how to breed zebrafish because this is something he knows. I'm not sure he knows why, he just does.

I'm sure he doesn't need to know why.

He spends his days staring at the frothy clusters of life-buoyed larvae stranded along the bottom of his standard-issue home aquarium. Once liberated from their capsules, these newbies are extremely hard to spot in their transparency.

Make no mistake: he can see them.

* * *

Zebrafish.

They are fairly ordinary with black stripes to justify the name. No galloping hooves, no long flowing tails, though the females have fins that look like the tails of silver horses in canter.

These aquatic pets are cheap to own, they spawn by the hundreds, and they grow quickly. What's even more useful is that, until they are adults, stripe or no stripe, they are transparent.

Scientists today keep tanks and tanks of hundreds of zebrafish to research drugs for neurological applications. Budgets for live foods like bloodworm and mosquito larvae have since become a regular part of Purchasing Department requisitions at research universities.

The scientists administer their experiments directly into the tanks where the zebrafish live and breed. I wonder if they use pipettes or just pour the contents of their media in like milk from a carton.

The fish don't seem to mind swimming in artificial baths of semi-water under close conditions, occasionally ending up in petri dishes and under microscopes where the curious watch and wait, tag and record.

Zebrafish are cheaper to breed and keep and can yield chemistry results far faster than mice and rats due to their accelerated growth cycles. A fat zebrafish female will spawn three hundred eggs outside her body, which are fertilized by males.

Mice usually have only eight pups.

One can infer how the hobby fish may eventually replace cages of lab mice in the basements of clinics, if only owing to the need for rapid consumption of test subjects.

The clear oyster-colored bubbles that house the embryos of zebrafish can develop myelin on their nerve cells by day 3 postpartum, along with bulging black eyes that are blind until the larvae pop, wriggling and spastic, from their hatches.

This is a modern miracle in biology.

So fast, so clear, so captive.

The fry remain transparent for weeks, growing rapidly: spines and tails and fins emerging in back-to-back cycles of metamorphosis. Acceleration to a cure? (For MS, for muscular dystrophy Duchenne, Alzheimer's?)

Maybe.

As many as 80 drugs per week can be tested using zebrafish embryos. Talk about fast track.

Why zebrafish matter to science is not a question the boy on YouTube can answer. The zebrafish shares three quarters of its genome with human beings. How ridiculous it might seem to assume any relationship between man and fish except for imaginary freaks like the Creature from the Black Lagoon or, maybe, Aquaman.

I wonder if the boy knows about the lost continent of Atlantis. He ought to.

* * *

For research into multiple sclerosis, the mouse model has been, for decades, the only way to test therapies.

As recently as 2017, a transgenic approach, which forces zebrafish to develop a kind of zoological MS mirror condition called EAE, was achieved. The lab rats may or may not be happy about this, since EAE has been the sword they've fallen on for generations.

But they should be relieved, at least. Using the zebrafish to test drugs for things like toxicity, dosage, and mechanisms of action first means the rodents will be spared the worst of the Frankensteinian failures.

I suppose the boy who keeps fish might also become the boy who adopts mice.

* * *

There is this problem of no answers when it comes to MS. MRI handed over some answers, which accelerated the journey to a cure back in the 1980s. Now, we can peek inside the brains of zebrafish, give them MS, and then—yes!—get rid of it!

Unlike human beings, zebrafish are neurologically resilient when it comes to remyelination. It's not all torture and genocide in the fingolimod** tank.

The future of animal research includes secure jobs in the field of zebrafish husbandry.

Maybe this will be the future of the YouTube boy. Maybe he will go from wobbly hand shots and too much voiceover to steward the protocol for colonizing his favorite pets using marbles and shallow water. He's already showed us his lifetime supply of dechlorination tablets.

Could today's third-grade hobby become tomorrow's cure for MS? I click *subscribe*.

Glia (est. 1988) is a peer-reviewed research journal devoted to studies of the structure and function of neuroglia.

**Fingolimod is one of several treatments used to curb or prevent demyelination in people with MS.*

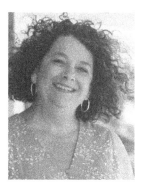

About the Author

Tamara Kaye Sellman wrote most of *Intention Tremor* next to a campfire or inside a travel trailer at Fort Worden State Park in Port Townsend, WA in the five years that followed her diagnosis of multiple sclerosis (MS) in June 2013.

A journalist by trade, she'd gone back to school to study sleep technology at age 47. While preparing for finals in March 2013, she discovered she could see, but she could no longer read. Other symptoms—especially tremors in her left leg and hands, balance and dizziness issues, chronic fatigue, deafening tinnitus, and sweeping sensations called *paresthesias*—still continue despite treatment.

Following diagnosis, Sellman finished the sleep technology program to earn two medical credentials (RPSGT, CCSH). After working overnight shift directly with patients for two years in the sleep lab, she now works as a science journalist, healthcare columnist for Health Union, and online community advocate.

She also serves as co-admin to the Multiple Sclerosis Unplugged Facebook group, is a member of both the education and content committees for the American Association of Sleep Technologists, contributes regularly to the magazine *A2Zzz*, and is a paid "influencer" for two of Healthline's chronic illness communities.

Her short work (essays, poems, stories, and articles) has been published widely and internationally. Sellman's work has been featured on postcards and calendars and inside city buses.

She's earned several awards including first place in the Dr. O. Marvin Lewis Essay Award and has been a finalist in contests sponsored by the Pacific Northwest Writers Association, the *North American Review*, *Winning Writers*, and others. Her creative nonfiction was nominated for the prestigious John S. Burroughs Prize. She's also received two Pushcart Prize nominations: one for fiction, the other for poetry.

Sellman writes across genres and forms, letting the work organically choose its final shape. Some of her work falls into multiple categories of prose and poetry, while other pieces may be described as hybrid. She is driven by the challenge to experiment and find surprising ways to approach universal themes. She delights in playing with forms as a way to unlock the themes she cares most about.

Besides MS and sleep medicine, Sellman enjoys writing about gardening, wildlife and the Pacific Northwest, often through a political lens. She currently lives in Kingston, WA.

Author proceeds from the sale of this book will be donated to the Accelerated Cure Project (https://www.acceleratedcure.org/). To donate, please visit their donation page at https://bit.ly/3cCbX9W.

CPSIA information can be obtained
at www.ICGtesting.com
Printed in the USA
FSHW011007191021
85491FS